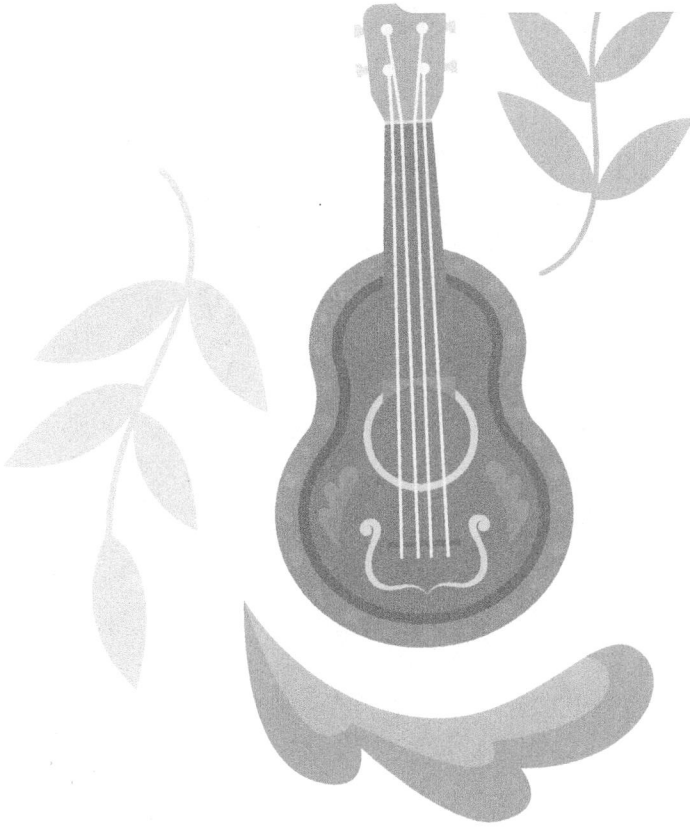

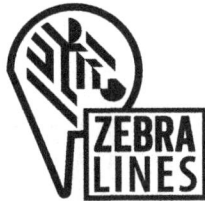

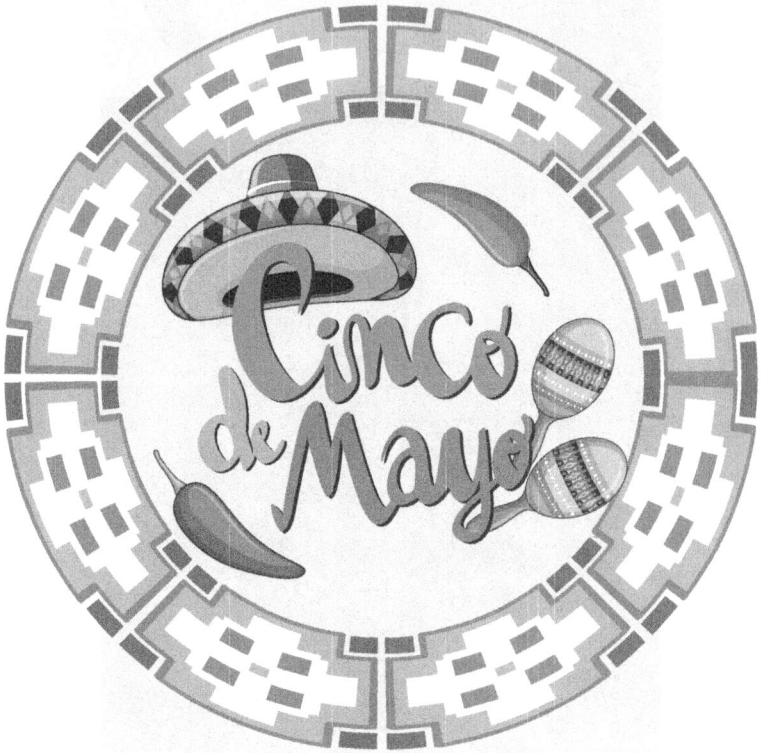

Cinco de Mayo

NOTEBOOK

SIMPLE TO-DO CHECKLIST WITH 3 TOP PRIORITIES

THIS BOOK BELONGS TO

MONTHLY TO-DO LIST

JANUARY

- [ ]
- [ ]
- [ ]
- [ ]
- [ ]

FEBRUARY

- [ ]
- [ ]
- [ ]
- [ ]
- [ ]

MARCH

- [ ]
- [ ]
- [ ]
- [ ]
- [ ]

APRIL

- [ ]
- [ ]
- [ ]
- [ ]
- [ ]

MAY

- [ ]
- [ ]
- [ ]
- [ ]
- [ ]

JUNE

- [ ]
- [ ]
- [ ]
- [ ]
- [ ]

JULY

- [ ]
- [ ]
- [ ]
- [ ]
- [ ]

AUGUST

- [ ]
- [ ]
- [ ]
- [ ]
- [ ]

SEPTEMBER

- [ ]
- [ ]
- [ ]
- [ ]
- [ ]

OCTOBER

- [ ]
- [ ]
- [ ]
- [ ]
- [ ]

NOVEMBER

- [ ]
- [ ]
- [ ]
- [ ]
- [ ]

DECEMBER

- [ ]
- [ ]
- [ ]
- [ ]
- [ ]

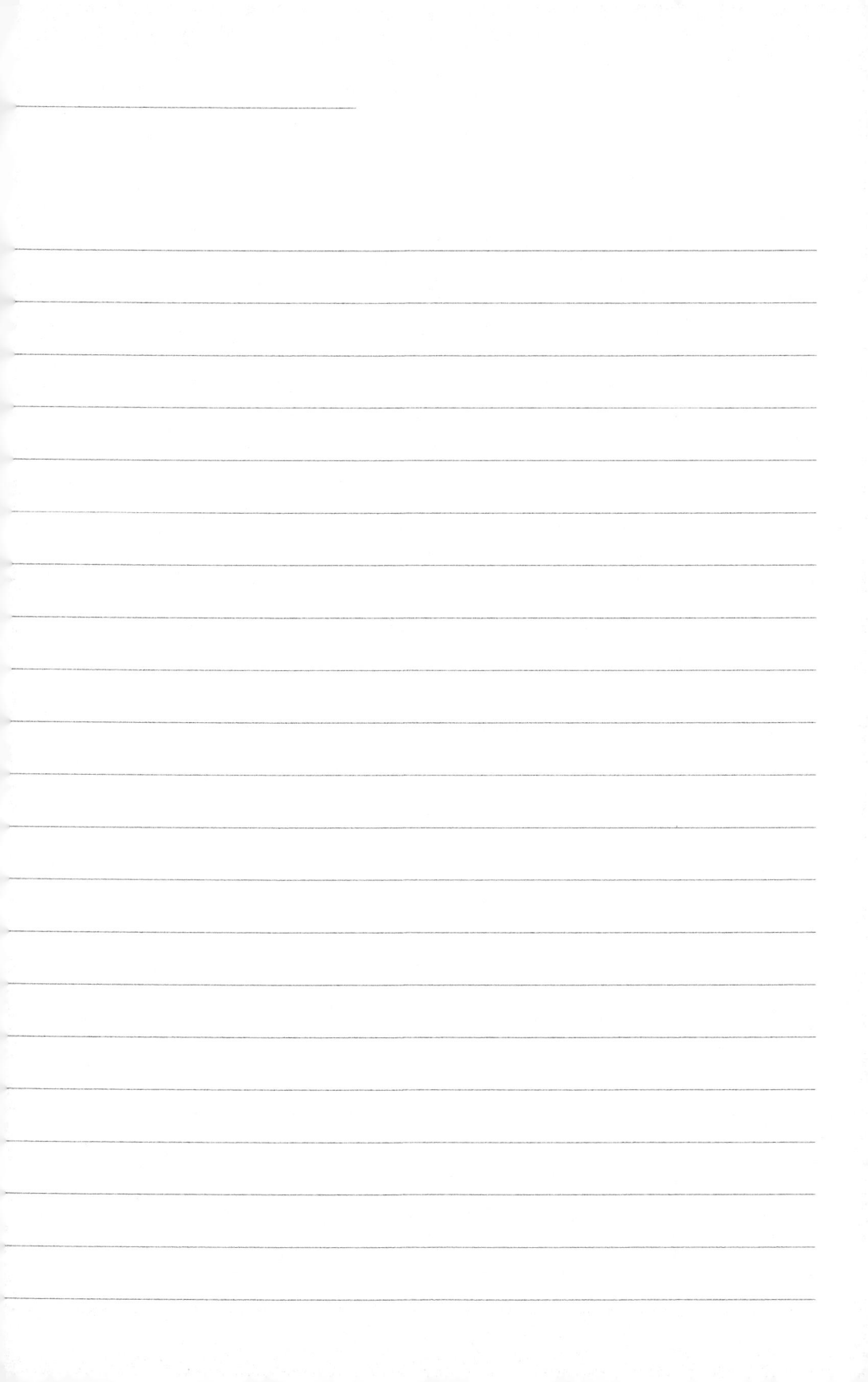

Date

Top Priority

1

2

3

LIST IT OUT

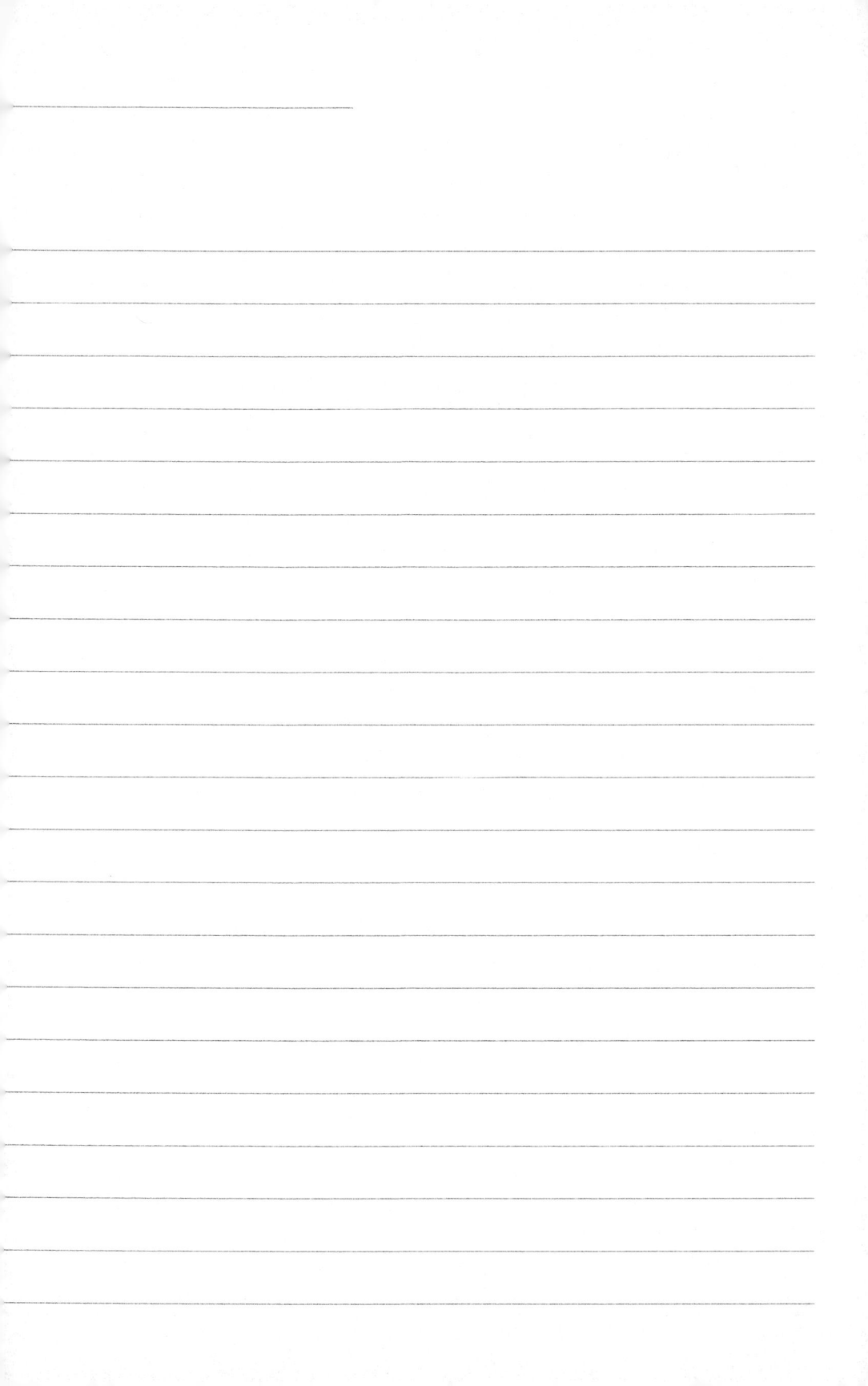

Date

Top Priority

1

2

3

LIST IT OUT

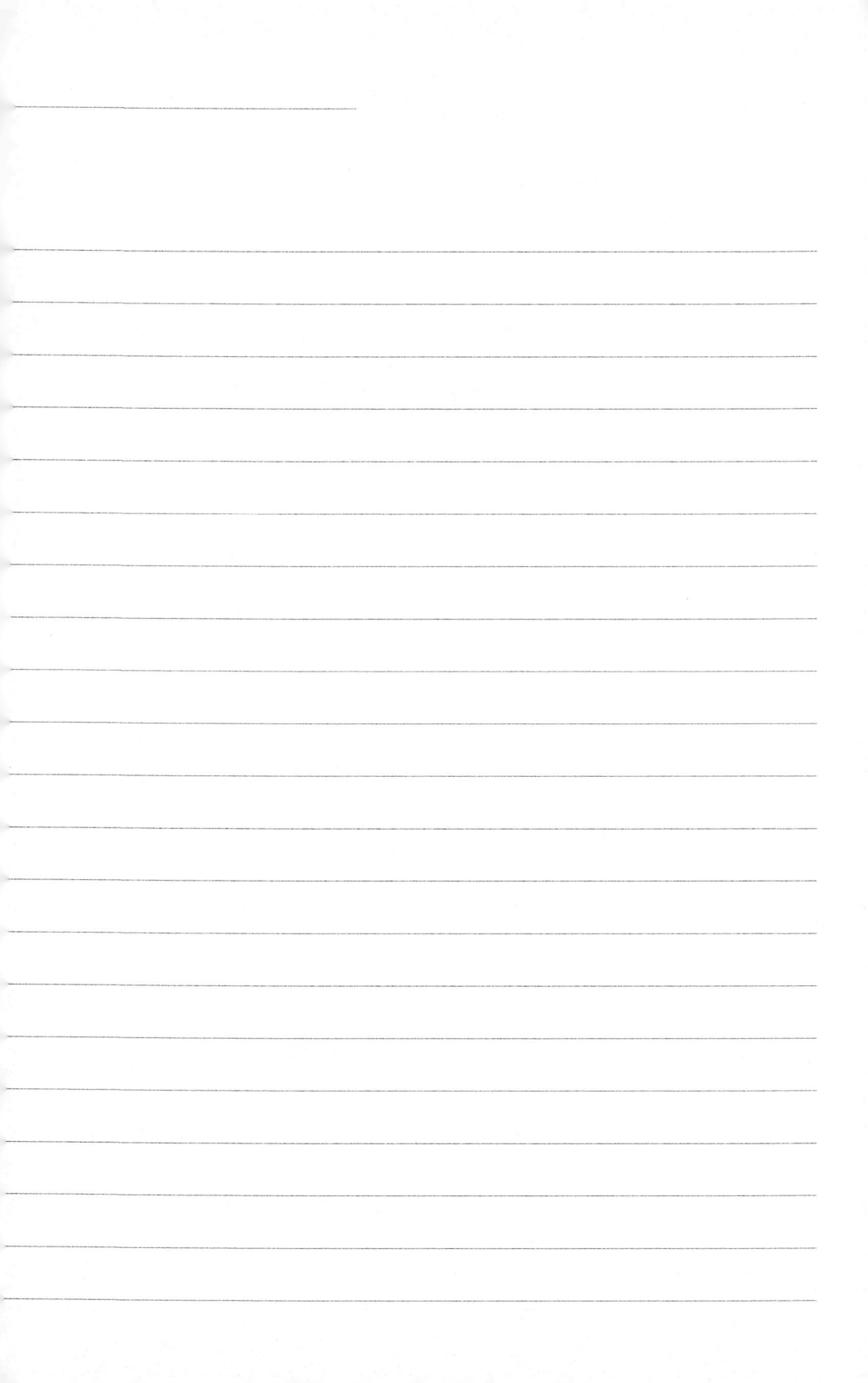

Date

Top Priority

1

2

3

LIST IT OUT

- _____
- _____
- _____
- _____
- _____
- _____
- _____
- _____
- _____
- _____
- _____
- _____
- _____
- _____

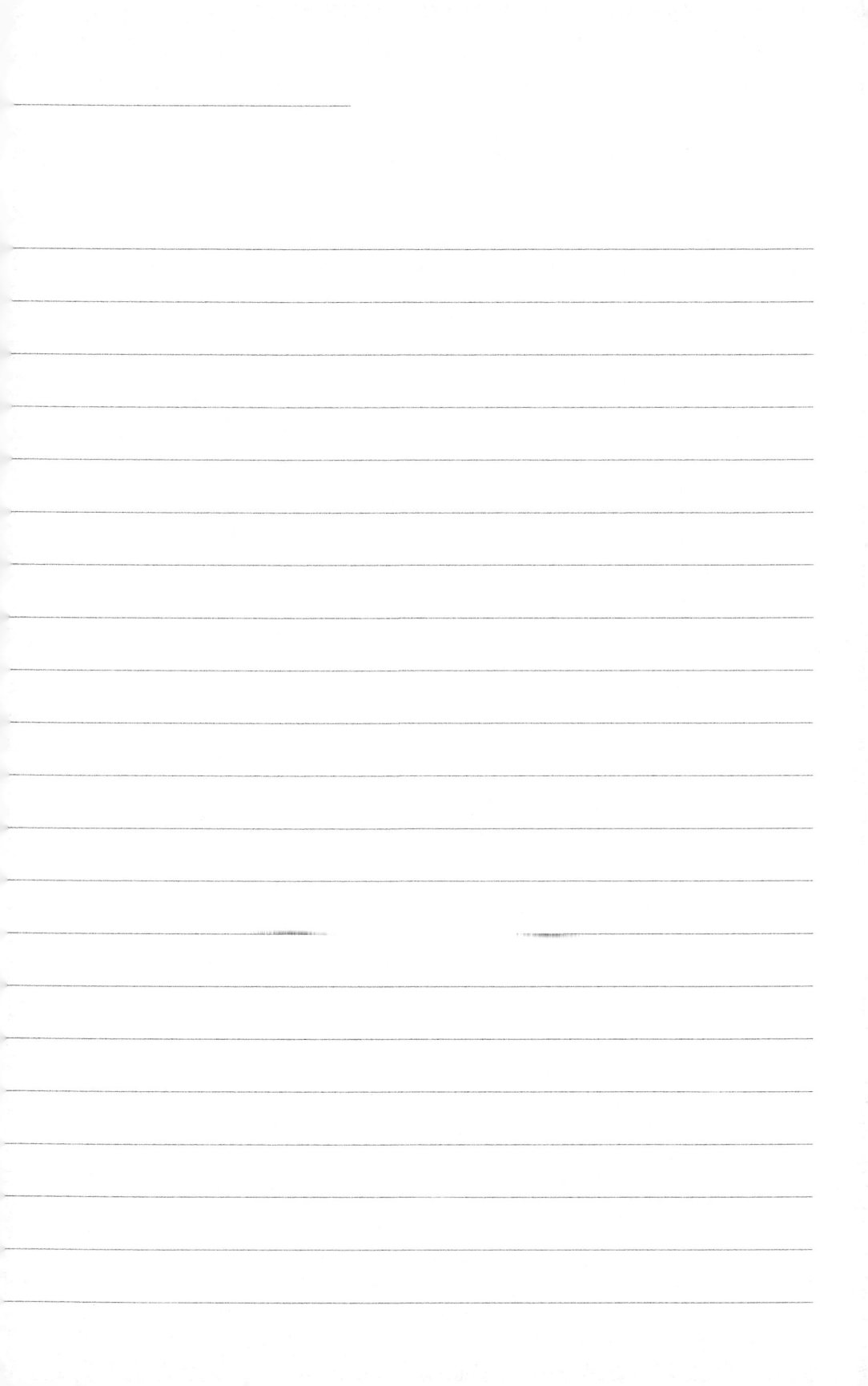

Made in the USA
Las Vegas, NV
08 May 2022